Worship & WELLNESS
• • • THE DISCOVERY • • •

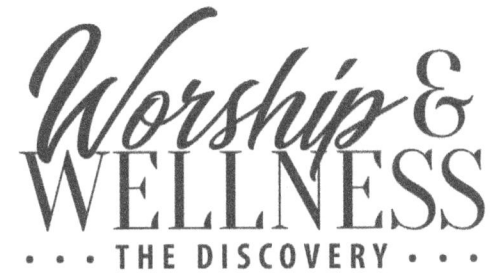

THE DISCOVERY

Seven Proven Strategies to Transform Your Temple

Oluchi Ibekwe Immanuel, MD

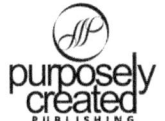

WORSHIP & WELLNESS
Published by Purposely Created Publishing Group™
Copyright © 2018 Oluchi Immanuel

All rights reserved.

No part of this book may be reproduced, distributed or transmitted in any form by any means, graphic, electronic, or mechanical, including photocopy, recording, taping, or by any information storage or retrieval system, without permission in writing from the publisher, except in the case of reprints in the context of reviews, quotes, or references.

Limit of Liability / Disclaimer of Warranty: While the publisher and author have used their best efforts in preparing this book, they make no representations or warranties with the respect to the accuracy or completeness of the contents of this book and specifically disclaim any implied warranties of fitness for a particular purpose. No warranty may be created or extended by sales representatives or written sales materials. The advice and strategies contained herein may not be suitable for your situation.

You should consult with a doctor where appropriate. Neither the publisher nor author shall be liable for any loss or damages including but not limited to special, incidental, consequential or other damages.

Printed in the United States of America
ISBN: 978-1-948400-45-9

Special discounts are available on bulk quantity purchases by book clubs, associations and special interest groups. For details email: sales@publishyourgift.com or call (888) 949-6228.

For information logon to:
www.PublishYourGift.com

Dedication

This book is dedicated to the love of my life. Kevin, you encouraged me when all I had to show for my passion was a far-fetched dream and some scribbles on a notepad. You are my confidant, you keep me laughing, and you are my "person." You are a dream come true. My love for you is indescribable.

I also dedicate this book to my darling children, being your mother has brought me more joy than I could have ever imagined. You inspire me to live my best health now and to help others on this wellness journey.

To my parents, brothers, sisters, nieces, nephews, and friends, thank you for the never-ending prayers, support, and encouragement.

Table of Contents

Introduction 1

CHAPTER 1
Recognize Who You Are in Christ 5

CHAPTER 2
Release Stress Through Wellness 15

CHAPTER 3
Realize It Is Not About Your Looks 27

CHAPTER 4
Reframe Your Thoughts 37

CHAPTER 5
Reclaim Your Health 47

CHAPTER 6
Reshape Your Nutrition Habits 57

CHAPTER 7
Restore Your Temple 65

CHAPTER 8
The Discovery 75

Thank You 79

Sources 81

About the Author 83

Introduction

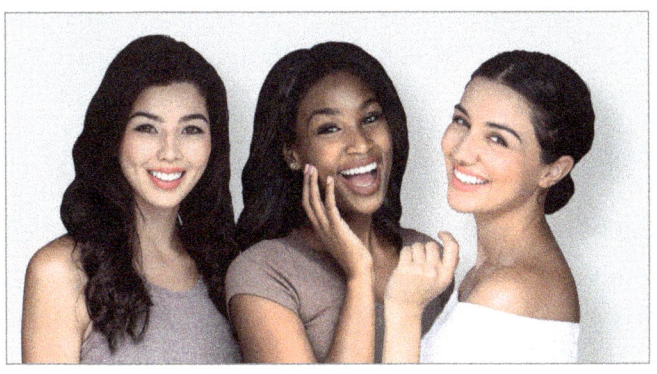

Beautiful Woman of God, this book is for you. I know the struggles you face balancing the many directions life seems to pull you in. I see your comments on social media in The Faith & Wellness Lifestyle Facebook group and your messages to @DrOluchiMD, and I get it. School is tough, work is demanding, friendships are trying, marriage can be a roller coaster, kids are clingy, family life is complicated, and the list goes on and on. Sometimes at the very bottom of this list, we manage to pencil in self-care. I know these struggles well, because, I too share them. Unfortunately, when self-care is placed so low on our list of priorities, other areas of our lives are affected as well. Consider this, as a plane is preparing for takeoff, the flight attendant usually says, "in the event of an emergency please place your mask on before helping others place their masks on." This may seem counterintuitive, but there is an important reason why these directions must be followed. If you are busy assisting others with their masks, before you put on your mask, you could faint due to lack of oxygen. At that point, *you cannot help anyone, including yourself.* In fact, now those who were depending on you for help, including children, will be *burdened with the stress* of figuring out how to help you. You cannot help yourself, much less others who need your love and care when you are not at your best. Conversely, when we intentionally take care of ourselves and prioritize our health and wellness—as women who are sisters, wives, daughters, and mothers—those around us greatly benefit as well.

In Worship and Wellness: The Discovery, we will examine God's will for our health and the true meaning of wellness. We will also explore the most common preventable chronic diseases and discuss practical ways to prevent or improve these conditions. Lastly, we will discover the incredible spiritual and physical benefits of fasting as a lifestyle.

Dear Sister, this book should be a gentle reminder to *put your mask on first.*

CHAPTER 1

Recognize Who You Are in Christ

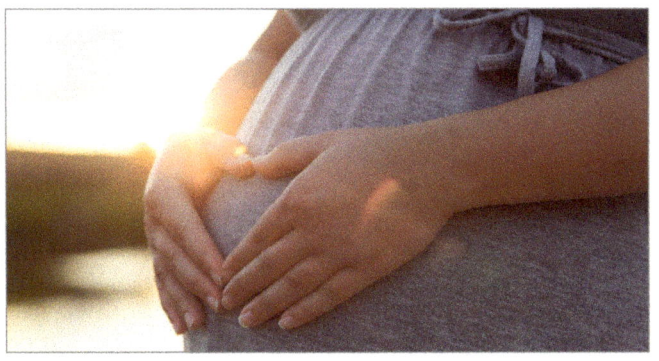

*"For you created my inmost being;
you knit me together in my mother's womb."*

(Psalms 139:13 New King James Version)

I have always been amazed by the process of gestation, from conception to the delivery of a baby. It all begins when millions of sperm are released, but only one makes it to the egg. Just twenty-four hours after fertilization the egg begins growing by rapidly dividing. Each step in the process is extremely detailed and requires exact precision, but a woman may not even know she is pregnant for several weeks. Yet God is there, knitting together the precious child in her womb. This is why no child is a mistake. There is no way this very complicated process could accidentally occur. God chose to knit you! And He did not just knit your physical features. He created your inner being, your personality, your temperament, your strengths, and your weaknesses.

In Psalms, David exclaims to God, *"You saw me before I was born. Every day of my life was recorded in your book. Every moment was laid out before a single day had passed." (Psalms 139:16 New Living Translation)* Even more incredible is that before God created you in your mother's womb, He *knew you* and *chose you*! *"Before I formed you in the womb*

I knew you, before you were born I set you apart; I anointed you as a prophet to the nations." (Jeremiah 1:5 New International Version)

Most of us can count on one hand the number of people in our lives who actually *know* us. We can put a mask on at work, at church and even with some family members, but not with God. He already knows. He knows the good and the bad. He knows your darkest secrets, your lowest points (He was there too), and the pain you feel when you remember those times. Remember, God has already seen every day that we have had, and those we are yet to experience, *before* we were created. He saw every heartache, every trial, every disappointment, every hurt, and every tear. He also saw the victories and the celebrations in your life. This is why it does not make sense to stress over any circumstance in life. God already knows how the situation will end, and He has promised that all things work out for our good in the end. If things do not seem to be working out for you, it is probably not the end or you may not yet understand the full situation. When my daughter was three years old, she owned a special coloring set consisting of markers and crayons, which she absolutely adored. One day, there was a special art event at her school and she insisted on bringing her coloring set. But when it was time to leave for the event, the coloring set was nowhere to be found. We searched every room in the house and all of her favorite hiding places. The coloring set was gone. My daughter was distraught. She cried and screamed and refused to go to the event without the coloring set. I tried to reassure her that she did not need the coloring set that night and we would find it when we returned but she was too upset to listen. I decided to give her some time and space to calm down. A few minutes later, she came to me with tears in her eyes and wrapped her arms around me. "I just want my colors" she whimpered. "I know" I replied while giving her a hug. "Let's go to school and we can continue to look for the coloring set when we get home." In my mind, there was absolutely no reason to cry over a set of old broken crayons and mostly dried out markers. My daughter did not know this but she was going to receive a brand new coloring set at the event. Reluctantly, she took my hand and we left for the event.

My daughter never looked for that old coloring set again once she got the new one. Sometimes we find ourselves in that same situation. We cry and scream about a job we feel we need or a relationship that ends sooner than we imagined. We try our best to hold on to the old, broken-down things in our lives when God has something much better waiting for us. No matter what situation we are facing, God has already seen the end. And, in the end *spoiler alert* WE WIN! So let us start trusting that God is in control. Let us take His hand and walk boldly in faith. This may seem easier to say than to do, but that is the essence of faith. Faith is jumping out of a plane and hoping that your parachute works. The first, and only time, I went skydiving, I remember being completely terrified while sitting in a tiny plane. I had always called myself a "thrill seeker." When I was younger, my older brother and I prided ourselves on researching the tallest and scariest roller coasters at every amusement park we visited, so we could conquer those rides at the beginning of our day. We never met a roller coaster we could not handle. And now here I was sitting in a plane thousands of miles above the ground with a tiny pouch on my back, shaking in fear. My brother was usually my support system for these "scary" events. When he was with me, I always knew I would be safe. It did not matter what we were doing, somehow I believed I could not get hurt when he was sitting next to me. Skydiving had always been on our "bucket list." However, I had not invited my brother on this adventure for a few reasons. First, the skydiving event was a last minute invitation from a friend of mine. And secondly if, God forbid, something went wrong I did not want my parents to feel even more heartache. I did, however, call my brother right before we took off. He prayed with me, "Lord, don't let her die!" He asked me several times if I was sure I wanted to do this and then he calmly told me I would be fine. His words were reassuring. As I sat in the plane contemplating my life, I decided at that moment I was not going to let fear hold me back from achieving any dream placed in my heart. Even if my main source of support was not present, I would still press on. When it was my turn to leave the plane, I looked down, closed my eyes and leaped! Thank God my parachute did work!

Faith is what God is requiring you to hold onto when it is time to jump. Let go of the old and embrace the new. He created you, He knows you and He loves you. Trust Him! Because guess what, despite all of your circumstances, God has called you to reach the nations! Your "nation" may look completely different from the woman next to you, but God has placed something within you that the world is waiting to know! In this day of social media, it is easier than ever to reach the world with a couple strokes of the keyboard. However, your "nation" could be your church ministry, the homeless shelter down the road, or an orphanage millions of miles away. The point is you have a mission that only you can accomplish. Have faith in the One, who knew you before you were created, to guide you to victory. And like any soldier, your body must be in the best shape to complete the task.

··· Pause & Reflect ···

1. What are three of your most unique qualities?

2. What is one situation in your life that you need to trust God to handle?

3. Who is your "nation?" What group of people would be blessed by your unique qualities and talents?

CHAPTER 2

Release Stress Through Wellness

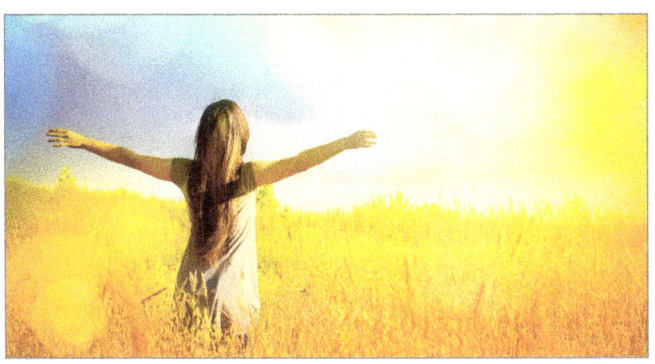

"Beloved, I pray that you may prosper in all things and be in health, just as your soul prospers."

(3 John 1:2 New King James Version)

It is 2 a.m. and you have just finished work or have finally gotten the baby back to sleep. You are exhausted. There are a hundred things still left on your to-do list. You toss and turn, thinking about your list, until 5 a.m. when you force yourself to get up and start another tiring day. Sound familiar? Dear Sister, the scene I just described is a recipe for disaster. Your body reacts negatively to stress especially when you are tired and overwhelmed. Did you know stress suppresses your immune system making you more vulnerable to sickness? Stress can cause symptoms such as headaches, difficulty sleeping, muscle pain, and stomach issues. Stress can also lead to high blood pressure, heart disease, diabetes and other chronic diseases. Also, stress causes the release of a hormone named cortisol, which can lead to excessive weight gain. Simply put, stress is not your friend, yet many of us live in a constant state of stress.

Stress can occur in many forms. There can be stress due to finances, relationships, school, work, children, health and much more. Usually, once we allow ourselves to get aggravated about one thing, the stress begins to build up like a snowball rolling down a hill. It is easy to stop a small snowball, but even a body builder would struggle to resist a large boulder of snow. Stress during emergency situations is a protective mechanism. If you are walking in a field and a large lion jumps out in front of you, you will immediately feel your heart pumping and your body beginning to sweat. The hormonal shift, and the resulting change in our body, is called the "fight or flight" response. Just as it states, your body is preparing you to either defend yourself against this wild beast or to run away to preserve your life. If we did not have this response to stressful situations, we would be less inclined to move quickly to protect ourselves from harm. The problem with stress is, as mentioned above, many of us live in a constant state of stress instead of occasional stress. Our minds are constantly mulling over the tasks we still need to accomplish, the paychecks that barely cover the bills, and our bosses that are demanding more and offering less. Often, we feel like we are holding up that boulder on our backs. This stress can lead to serious health problems. It can be difficult to see how to get away from the stress.

When I was in medical school, I vividly remember basically living in our Learning Resource Center (LRC), which was the student library. Most days I was there for at least sixteen hours and during test weeks, I found myself in the LRC for up to twenty hours. I was beyond stressed. Every night I would dream about whatever topic I had read the day before and I would wake up feeling even more mentally exhausted than when I had gone to sleep. My eating habits were terrible and I was snacking on excessive amounts of sugar to make it through the day. I gained a significant amount of weight during that period of time and my personal life suffered, as I did not have time or energy to maintain my friendships. I knew if I did not make some changes quickly, I had the potential to spiral out of control. But for the grace of God. I thank God that through that season, He kept me grounded. I attended a great church, received frequent prayer and encouraging calls from my parents, and I was blessed with great friends who were going through the struggle with me. Also, I met the love of my life just as I was beginning to see the light at the end of the tunnel. Most importantly, in that season, I learned how to hear from God in the Valley. That would not be the last stressful period of my life. If you are familiar with medical training, you know that Residency made medical school seem like a walk in the park. Nonetheless, the truths I learned during that season of my life have continued to guide me. Let me share a few of those pearls with you.

The way to take back control of your life and free yourself from stress is to pursue a life of wellness. So, what is wellness? Wellness is comprised of three main components: mind, body, and soul. Many of us have the soul part covered, we love Jesus and we have a relationship with Him. However, you cannot live in complete wellness without the other two components, mind and body. In the Bible, the author of 3 John 1:2 desired that his loved ones would prosper in health just as their souls prosper. This was not to say the body is as important as our spiritual health, but rather to say physical health should be a close second. See, you cannot complete all God has called you to do if you are not living your best health. You may be called to share your anointed voice with the masses, but if you are constantly out of breath from being overweight or out of shape, you are limiting what you are able to achieve.

The "Parable of the Talents," in Matthew 25:14-30, tells of a master going on a journey and entrusting his property to three of his servants before leaving. The parable goes on to describe how each servant was given a different amount of talents. When the master returned, each servant was called on to give an account of what they did with the talent given. The master was pleased with the servants who took their talents and immediately put them to work to make more talents. However, the master was furious with the third servant who hid his talent in the ground. In fact, the master ordered that the third servant's talents be given to the first servant who had done well! We can consider our health to be like the talents given to each of the servants. Some of us have a harder time than others losing weight, some have genetic health conditions, and some have disabilities which make it more difficult to stay healthy. However, we have all been given some measure of health and we will be held accountable for what we choose to do with our health. There is a common saying that "health is wealth." This statement is true because your health is your most valuable possession. It does not matter how much money you have in the bank, if you are too ill to enjoy it, it is of no use to you. Like any financial investor would say, the key to building and maintaining wealth is to consistently make wise investments. For example, if you had purchased one thousand shares of Amazon in the initial days, you would be a millionaire today. Likewise, we can make small daily investments in our health that can lead to great future gains. One of the best examples of investing in your health is to quit smoking. Smoking is one of the leading causes of premature death in the United States and this is mostly due to heart disease. However, just minutes after the last cigarette is smoked, the person begins reaping major health benefits, which extend for years. Approximately fifteen years after quitting, the person likely has the same risk of heart disease as someone who never smoked. That's incredible! Other daily health investments with great rewards are improving our diets and exercising regularly.

We have been given the special gift of health. Therefore, we must learn to be good stewards of our health. When we take care of our bodies, we bring joy to God. God sees this as a pleasing sacrifice. *"Don't you realize that your body is the temple of the Holy Spirit, who lives in you and was given to you by God? You do not belong to yourself, for God bought you with a high price. So you must honor God with your body." (1 Corinthians 6:19-20 New Living Translation)*

The last part of the wellness triad is the mind. You must achieve peace of mind to be able to live a stress-free life. Your mind is a powerful tool. Your mind shapes the way you interact with the world. Did you know technically we see with our minds? Our eyes transmit details of colors, shapes, and other visual cues to the brain and then the brain decides what we see and what to do with the information. Think about the analogy of the glass filled to the halfway point with water. Some people will automatically see the glass as "half full" with plenty of opportunities to fill it to the top. Others will see the glass as "half empty" and may feel discouraged or disadvantaged. However, remember it is the SAME GLASS. Learning how to frame your mindset is an important key to succeeding in life. We will discuss more about this topic in the upcoming chapters. Being successful in your health, relationships, work, etc.--it all starts with your mind. *"Set your minds on things above, not on earthly things." (Colossians 3:2 New International Version)*

··· Pause & Reflect ···

1. What are some areas in which you are feeling stressed out or overwhelmed?

\
\
\
\

2. What are practical ways you can be a better steward of your health?

a) How can you pursue wellness in your everyday life?

CHAPTER 3

Realize It Is Not About Your Looks

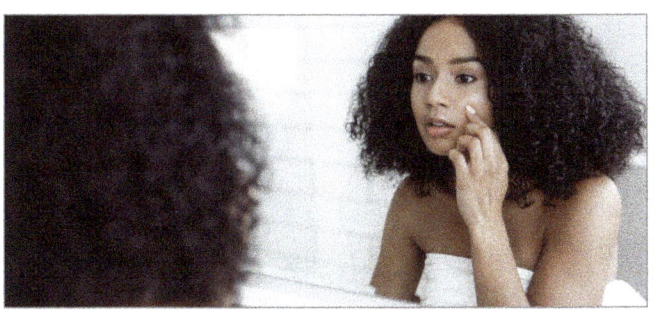

"So God created mankind in His own image, in the image of God He created them; male and female He created them."

(Genesis 1:27 New International Version)

It is not hard to figure out what the world considers "beautiful." We see billboards, magazine photos, movies and Instagram posts with women of a certain size and certain features. It seems that Hollywood has set a standard that women either try to achieve or may feel rejected because they feel they cannot meet those standards. But God has set His own standard for us. And guess what? It is not about your looks. How could it be about your looks when you were created in His image? You are already the epitome of beauty. *"For we are God's masterpiece. He has created us anew in Christ Jesus, so we can do the good things He planned for us long ago." (Ephesians 2:10 New Living Translation)"* God is much less worried about what is on the outside, than what is on the inside. Society will tell you to do whatever it takes to get followers and likes. As a physician, I have seen it all from waist trainers, to cleanses, to inversion hair growth challenges. People will spend hours and countless dollars to improve their outer bodies. Women can find four hours to sit at a hair salon but cannot fit in a 30-minute exercise session. We spend time and energy worrying about the wrong things! I once took care of a patient who had a heart condition that required a surgical procedure as treatment. The patient had come to my office because she refused to have the surgery. My patient was a beautiful middle-aged woman who was wearing a perfectly tailored suit and matching heels. When I asked her why she did not want the surgery, she explained that she was concerned about how the pacemaker would look in her chest and how obvious the scar might appear. She was willing to risk a life-threatening event because treatment of the condition could lead to a scar. All I could do was counsel her about the risks and benefits of the surgery. What I really wanted to say was, "this minor imperfection could save your life." We need to focus on what truly matters. Have you ever picked up a beautiful, shiny apple and bit into it only to find that the inside is rotten? You can clean the apple as much as you want, but if the inside is decaying, the apple is not suitable to be eaten. Ladies, your health deserves more attention than your outer beauty. Let's work on improving our health first. Interestingly, most people find when you work on the inside--improving your eating habits, sleep, exercise, etc.—your outer appearance also reflects these beneficial changes. For example, fruits and vegetables can contain nutrients and antioxidants that give your skin a natural glow. And sleeping seven to eight hours each day can improve your energy and decrease the puffiness under your eyes.

When discussing healthier lifestyle habits, the topic that always comes to the forefront is weight loss. I understand that this is a painful topic for some people. Many women have been tormented, bullied or shamed because of their weight. Some have been denied jobs, promotions or have been rejected by people in their personal lives who could not see past their weight to get to know them. Others have struggled year after year with various diets and have felt hopeless when the number on the scale remained the same. I want you to know that I see you and I understand your pain. I am sorry our society is so obsessed with weight in terms of appearances but not health. I am also sorry if your doctor has tried to talk to you about your weight in a way that you found condescending or hurtful. The medical community is trying to improve the way we talk about obesity or being overweight, but we still have a long way to go. So, let's look at what is a healthy weight. The Body Mass Index (BMI) formula is the most common tool used to determine whether or not a person is at a healthy weight. This formula calculates a measurement of body mass based on height and weight, and then gives a value called the BMI. Based on the value, your BMI places you in the underweight, normal weight, overweight or obesity category. The calculator is not perfect, however, it provides a good starting point when assessing one's health. Obesity as a medical condition is not something we can sweep under the rug. Being obese drastically increases your risk of chronic conditions (more than being overweight) and it can even shorten your lifespan. We now know that obesity is not a lack of will power, it is a serious medical condition that can be caused by hormonal imbalances. Obesity should be addressed and treated just as any other chronic medical condition such as diabetes. I recently read an article about a woman who felt offended when her doctor brought up her weight during a medical visit for an unrelated condition. Let me tell you something Sister, if you are overweight or obese and your doctor does NOT discuss your weight during any visit, then your doctor is doing you a disservice. People rarely come to see their Primary Care Physicians to discuss their weight, but doctors must use any opportunity to let you know about the possible negative consequences of obesity. We will talk more about chronic medical conditions such as obesity in this book. I ask that you read the words with an open heart. Release the hurt and focus on the freedom a truly healthy lifestyle can bring you.

Let me also point out, to the naturally skinny Sisters who feel none of this applies to them—just because your weight is normal, does not necessarily mean that you are healthy. You cannot automatically know the state of a person's health just by looking at his or her outer appearance. Unfortunately, I have diagnosed many patients with type 2 diabetes who were in the "normal" weight category. Diet, family history, and lack of exercise are some of the other factors that can play a role in the development of type 2 diabetes. There are areas of health we could all stand to work on, so let us not be quick to judge.

"But the LORD said to Samuel, 'Do not consider his appearance or his height, for I have rejected him. The LORD does not look at the things people look at. People look at the outward appearance, but the LORD looks at the heart.'"

(1 Samuel 16:7 New International Version)

··· Pause & Reflect ···

1. What does "being beautiful" mean to you?

2. What value do you place on inner vs. outer beauty? And why?

3. How do you feel about your weight? What is your BMI?

CHAPTER 4
Reframe Your Thoughts

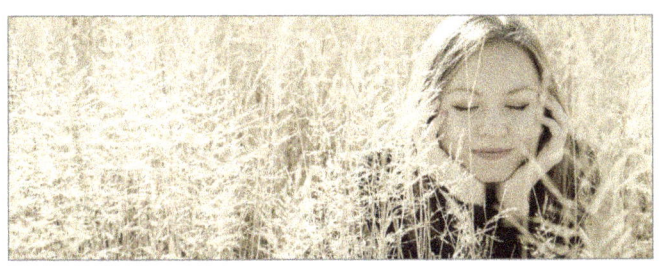

"Keep this Book of the Law always on your lips; meditate on it day and night, so that you may be careful to do everything written in it. Then you will be prosperous and successful."

(Joshua 1:8 New International Version)

Webster's dictionary defines the word meditate as "to engage in mental exercise (such as concentration on one's breathing or repetition of a mantra) for the purpose of reaching a heightened level of spiritual awareness." In Joshua Chapter 1, the children of God were instructed to meditate on the Law "day and night" to become "prosperous and successful." Essentially, you will become what you focus all of your mental energy on. You will achieve a high level of spiritual awareness and have success in whatever God has instructed you to do when you meditate on the promises of God and what God has said about your life. Conversely, our minds can also place limits on our lives without us even realizing it. I once heard a story about a cricket that was caught by a child and placed in a cup with the lid on it. The cricket jumped all night trying to escape from the cup. Each time it jumped, it would hit its head on the lid of the cup. The next day the cricket continued to jump, but it no longer jumped as high. Now it would only jump to right under the level of the lid so that it would not hit its head. Eventually, the child was able to remove the lid and the cricket would not even try to escape because it had been conditioned to only jump to a certain level, *despite having the full capability to jump much higher.* A similar phenomenon can be seen in circus elephants. Elephants are the largest land animals. They can grow to thirteen feet tall and weigh up to 14,000 pounds. Yet, at a circus, it is not uncommon to see an elephant being bound by a simple chain around its leg connected to a peg in the ground. How does this happen? It starts early in the elephant's life. When the elephant is a baby, a strong rope is placed around its leg to keep it from escaping. Naturally, the baby elephant will fight the rope with all of its strength. The elephant pushes and pulls and struggles, sometimes enduring pain along the way, until the elephant finally realizes that it cannot escape. From that moment on the elephant stops trying. Even when it grows two or three times larger, that same tiny rope is able to keep the elephant bound. *The mighty elephant has become trapped, not by the situation and not by the rope, but by its own thoughts.*

My Sister, your life will radically change if you can grasp this very truth and internalize it. Our own thoughts and mental blocks can prevent us from getting to the next step in life, whether it is achieving health goals, closing a deal, starting a business, joining a ministry and so on. Think back to your childhood, what negative things were you told that you have held on to? I remember a teacher telling me she would "never go to a black doctor." Another teacher told me I would not be accepted into any college, because I dropped her typing class, despite my 4.4 GPA. I thank God that my parents encouraged me to shoot for the moon. Whenever I complained that something was too hard, my Nigerian parents would reply "Are you the first to do it? Do the other people have two heads?" And then they would remind me I could do all things through Christ even if I were the first person to do it. As immigrants, my parents know firsthand what it is like to have all the odds stacked against you. They arrived in this country with little more than some change in their pockets and the clothes in their suitcases. Yet, they *saw* the life they wanted for themselves and their kids and did not let anything keep them from achieving their goals. This highlights my next point.

You need to see yourself having already won. What goal are you striving to achieve at this moment? What will be your first reaction when you achieve this goal? Will you cry, scream, or dance? Who will be the first person you call? What will you say? How will you celebrate? Where will you go? What will you order? What clothing will you be wearing? How will you style your hair? What shoes will you be wearing? These are the types of questions that you should be able to answer about each of your goals. You are literally building the framework in your mind so all that is left is to step into it. This is your mindset. Remember, we see with our minds. If you cannot see yourself victorious, how do you expect anyone else to? You must eliminate the thoughts that are holding you back. Remove your mental ropes and chains so you can see visions of success. You must change your mindset. So how do you do this? First, start by taking inventory of your thoughts. Take some time to journal every day. Write your reflections and feelings down, whether it is a few sentences or a few pages, make sure you capture your emotions. This process will allow you to identify areas you should focus on.

The next step is to empower yourself with scripture and affirmations. Affirmations are positive thoughts and language used to generate and create the desired outcome. An affirmation is "seeing" your victory. Whenever a negative thought enters your mind, cancel it with a positive affirmation. For example, you may think you are not strong enough to change your eating habits. You can replace that negative thought with the following affirmation: "God has equipped me with the strength to overcome any obstacle before me." You should say your affirmations aloud and write them down. When I was applying to medical school, I did not have the guidance or support I needed from my University. I attended a large school and the pre-medical support staff, at that time, was not well equipped to guide students in the application process. At one point, I was forced to choose between a medical school interview and retaining my research grant. In addition, I struggled with the MCAT exam, receiving high scores on the practice tests, and then scoring slightly lower on the actual exam. I felt discouraged by the application process. I began to doubt myself. I even considered taking a year off from school and applying with the next cycle. However, I felt God urging me to trust Him. He was the One who put the desire in my heart to help people live healthier lives. By that point, I had already completed a research program helping African American women stop smoking and I was in the process of another project studying obesity in young kids. I knew without a doubt that this was what I was called to do! I began to pray specifically about the application process. I prayed for wisdom, guidance and favor. I also asked my prayer group at church and my parents to pray for me as well. I began envisioning myself as a doctor. I could see myself examining patients and diagnosing medical conditions. I could see myself empowering my patients to take control of their health. I even purchased a white coat and had my friend take a picture of me, which I captioned "looking into the future." My mindset had completely changed. I still have that picture. Every time I look at it, it reminds me of the importance of seeing myself having already won the battle. I went on to apply to medical school that year. Not only did I get accepted, I was accepted to ten medical schools! I decided to choose my top school and I also received a scholarship. I went from feeling inadequate to having several options. It was truly a testimony of God's goodness in my life. However, I would not have been in the position to receive this blessing if I had not changed my mindset. It is in our control to adjust our mindset no matter what the circumstances are around us. Remember, you were chosen. You were called. God created you for a purpose. Don't let any mental blocks keep you from achieving your purpose. Change your mindset. *"For 'who has known the mind of the LORD that he may instruct Him?' But we have the mind of Christ." (1 Corinthians 2:16 New King James Version)*

··· Pause & Reflect ···

1. What are the three most important goals you are working towards at this moment? Paint a picture of your victory with each goal.

_____

_____

_____

_____

_____

2. What mindset block is holding you back?

_____

_____

_____

_____

_____

3. What are three Scriptures and affirmations you can use to address the mindset block?

CHAPTER 5

Reclaim Your Health

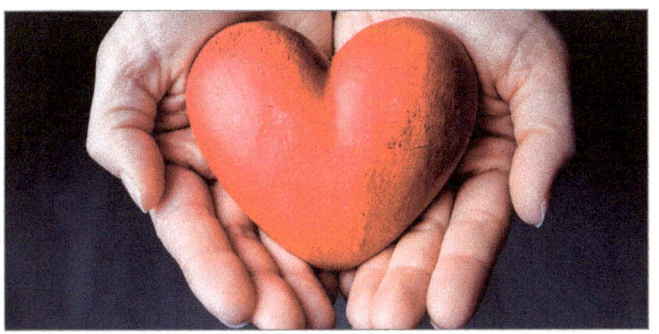

"Behold, I will bring to it health and healing, and I will heal them; I will reveal to them an abundance of peace and truth."

(Jeremiah 33:6 New American Standard Bible)

I once had a patient who was a very sweet lady in her late sixties. She would give me a big hug each visit and tell me how much I reminded her of her daughter. We had the same conversation each visit. I would say, "Mrs. X, your glucose levels are getting higher. Have you started cutting back on your sugar and carbohydrates? Did you fill that prescription that I gave you?" Without fail, she would always respond, "Now you know I'm not claiming that diabetes thing. I've been praying about it every day." We would sit and talk and I would try my best to explain how we still needed to treat the condition while she prayed. Unfortunately, Mrs. X declined to treat her diabetes and eventually developed kidney disease requiring dialysis three days each week. My heart aches every time I think about her. Sadly, her story is not unique. I have seen many patients with similar experiences due to untreated medical conditions. Now I am a firm believer in praying and trusting God to heal. After all, God is Jehovah Rapha, as He introduced Himself in Exodus 15. The word "rapha" means to heal, to cure or to restore. God proclaimed that He is our healing. This is not for a particular disease or condition, God simply is healing. Therefore, we do not get to choose HOW God will heal. God may choose to heal you through medication or through an operation or He can heal you with divine intervention. We all hope and pray for the latter but it is not up to us to choose. God may answer your prayers by directing you to a particular doctor who He will use to bring you to health. Imagine a person getting to Heaven and asking God why He did not send a healing, only to hear God say "I provided you with healthy foods and the ability to exercise to prevent this condition. Then I sent you medications to manage the disease and you still did not accept them." What a tragedy that would be. My prayer is that no one hears those words.

Disease prevention is the best strategy for living a healthy life. However, most people do not realize that staying healthy takes effort! Just like having a well-functioning car requires maintenance checks, oil changes, tire rotations, and much more, living a healthy life also requires some work. Let's take a look at a few of the most common preventable chronic diseases.

Hypertension or high blood pressure is a condition that occurs when the pressure within your arteries rises, making it more difficult for your heart to pump blood. Imagine a water hose with a kink in it. The pressure in the hose rises as water continues to flow and the hose will eventually explode due to the pressure. In medical terms, that is called a hemorrhagic stroke, which we will discuss later, and it is an unfortunate complication of hypertension. The cause of hypertension is multifactorial, meaning a number of things can cause a person's blood pressure to remain elevated. *You may be at risk for hypertension if you have a family history of hypertension, are overweight, are under stress or if you have a diet high in sodium.* Hypertension is known as the "silent killer" because most people do not have symptoms until their blood pressure is dangerously elevated.

Diabetes is a condition that occurs when there is a problem with a hormone called insulin. There are many types of diabetes, however, we will focus on type 2 because this particular type is preventable. Type 2 diabetes occurs when a person's body becomes resistant to insulin. Your body is making enough insulin and in some cases too much, but the insulin is unable to do its job. The role of insulin is to take glucose, which is sugar, from the bloodstream and transfer it into the cells where it can be used for energy or stored as fat. In type 2 diabetes, the insulin does not work properly which leaves high levels of glucose in the bloodstream. Over time, the high levels of glucose start to damage the small arteries in the body. This can cause heart disease, blindness, kidney failure and nerve damage. All of these conditions can lead to increased risk of death. *You may be at risk for type 2 diabetes if you are overweight, have a family history of diabetes, have hypertension, or if you have low levels of physical activity.*

Osteoarthritis is another common chronic condition. Arthritis is a broad term for inflammation of the joints and can have many causes. Osteoarthritis is arthritis caused by overuse or "wear and tear" of the joints. This type is most commonly associated with obesity. Being overweight places additional stress on the joints, as well as possibly causing an inflammatory response in the non-weight-bearing joints. *For every one pound a person is overweight, at least four pounds of additional pressure is exerted on the weight-bearing joints.* For example, a woman who is twenty pounds overweight has an extra eighty pounds of weight exerted on her hips and knees. This can cause chronic joint damage.

Cardiovascular diseases, meaning of the heart and blood vessel, can also be preventable conditions. Some examples of cardiovascular diseases are heart attacks and strokes. A heart attack occurs when there is a blockage in a blood vessel that supplies the heart. The particular part of the heart muscle that is not getting blood flow and oxygen begins to die. If this is not reversed quickly, a large enough portion of the heart muscle could be affected which can lead to death. A stroke occurs when there is either a blockage in a vessel in the brain (ischemic) or a bleeding vessel in the brain (hemorrhagic). Various parts of the body can be drastically affected post-stroke since the brain is the control center of the body. *A person can be at risk of cardiovascular diseases if he or she is overweight, a smoker,* *has poor nutrition, has low levels of physical activity or has been diagnosed with conditions such as diabetes and hypertension.*

You may have noticed there is one condition that is a common risk factor for all of the preventable medical conditions that were named above. This condition is obesity.

Obesity is a serious medical condition, which deserves the same type of focused evaluation and treatment as any other medical condition. Obesity is not just some extra weight, it is a complex disease that is caused by changes in hormone levels throughout the body. Unfortunately, the number of people who are overweight or obese throughout the world is increasing each year. There is now even a subspecialty of medicine that focuses specifically on obesity. The good news about obesity is it can be reversed and losing weight almost immediately reduces the risks associated with being overweight. There are many factors associated with the development of obesity, however, the most common are diet and family history. We will discuss practical solutions to addressing obesity in the next couple chapters.

··· Pause & Reflect ···

1. What role does faith play in how you view health/ healing?

2. What medical conditions are common in your family?

3. What are you doing to prevent chronic medical conditions?

CHAPTER 6
Reshape Your Nutrition Habits

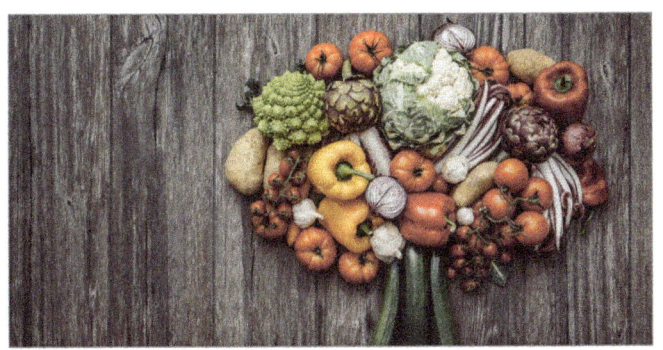

"For life is more than food, and the body more than clothes."

(Luke 12:23 New International Version)

It's Thanksgiving Day, the family is gathered, the decorations are up and the mood is festive. Everyone is waiting for one thing. The FOOD. Whether it's turkey, ham, green beans, pecan pie or macaroni and cheese, food is on everyone's mind. In fact, most people cannot think of Thanksgiving without food. Food has been ingrained in our culture and we expect food at most events. Can you imagine attending a conference or a wedding without food? Now food, in itself, is not the problem. The constant consumption of foods high in sugar or processed components is the problem. The further we get away from plant-based whole foods, the worse the obesity epidemic becomes. Food is intended to provide nourishment. Instead, we use food to fulfill other roles such as emotional support (ice cream after a depressing date) and entertainment (can't watch a movie without popcorn). The physiology of food, meaning the way food affects the body on a cellular level, is very interesting. Specific hormones are released when we eat certain foods and this makes us feel good. These are the same hormones released when a drug addict takes drugs and an alcoholic has a drink. Therefore, it is not surprising that food can be addicting. Also, different foods trigger our "fullness" hormones in different ways. For example, you could easily drink a large fountain soda without feeling full for more than a few minutes, but if you were to eat a steak, similar in calories, you would more than likely feel full for several hours. This is why calories are not all equal. Living in wellness means learning about healthy foods and changing your diet to achieve a healthier lifestyle.

Knowing exactly what you are eating is a good place to start. This is why it is important to look at the food labels on every single piece of food you eat. You should understand what the numbers truly mean when you read food labels. For example, if a label says the serving size is two pieces and there are ten servings per pack, the number of carbohydrates listed is only accurate if you eat two pieces. You need to calculate the correct amount of carbohydrates if you eat more. So why do those numbers matter? The number of carbohydrates is important because there are recommended amounts of the food components (nutrients) needed and this amount should not be exceeded, especially if you are working on losing weight. Some studies indicate obesity is associated with the "insulin theory" which explains how foods that lead to elevated levels of insulin are more likely to cause weight gain. According to this theory, eating foods with lower glycemic indexes will lead to lower insulin levels and thus weight loss. Many studies are showing this theory to be superior to the previously embraced "calorie in, calorie out" theory of weight loss. The calorie in, calorie out theory explains that the only way to lose weight is to eat a smaller amount of calories than you burn off each day. This theory is inherently flawed, however, because we know that eating one thousand calories of broccoli each day is not the same as eating one thousand calories of ice cream daily.

Although it may seem nutrition recommendations, like what percentage of your diet should be fats, are constantly changing, focusing on a few key points will greatly improve the quality of your diet. An improved diet and nutritional plan will lead to better health. The key points to focus on are:

1. Increase your intake of vegetables.

2. Eat a low to moderate amount of fruit daily.

3. If you choose to eat meat, keep the amount low to moderate and also choose the best quality available (i.e., grass-fed).

4. Remove sodas and sugary drinks from your diet.

5. Cut out sugary snacks from your diet.

6. Reduce your carbohydrate intake to low or moderate.

7. Increase your water and fiber intake.

These seven healthy diet changes combined with exercise can improve your health and overall quality of life. Exercise is especially important for women over the age of forty because women begin to lose muscle mass and gain weight around this age. Starting a daily exercise regimen with resistance exercises can help to prevent muscle loss.

··· Pause & Reflect ···

1. What role does nutrition play in your health?

2. What are some areas of your diet that could use improvement?

3. How can you start making these changes today?

CHAPTER 7
Restore Your Temple

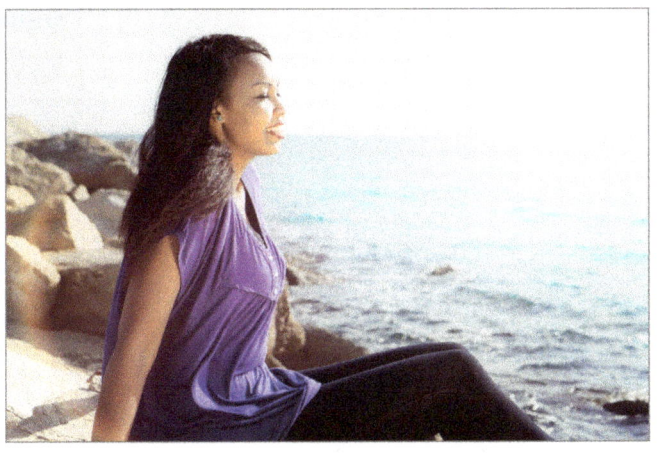

"He told them, "This kind can come out only by prayer and fasting."

(Mark 9:29 International Standard Version)

Most people look for a diet that will lead to fast results when they decide they want to lose weight. There are hundreds of different diets out there. Diets are binding, strict methods of forcing you to eat in a particular way. There are juicing diets, ketogenic diets, Mediterranean diets, fat burner diets, paleo diets, and the list goes on. While some people may see results from these diets, diets, in general, are hard to maintain for more than a short period of time. So how can you achieve weight loss in a way that is not stressful and is easy to maintain as a lifestyle? Consider intermittent fasting as a wellness game changer! Specifically going without food, while staying well hydrated with water, for a predetermined amount of time. Fasting has been around since the beginning of time. It is mentioned throughout the Bible, from Esther in the Old Testament, to Jesus in the New Testament. There are incredible spiritual benefits from fasting. Is there a problem or situation in your life you have been praying about but have not yet seen results? Try fasting. In Mark 9:29, Jesus' disciples were in a similar situation and Jesus' response was simple, "this kind can come out by nothing but prayer and fasting." Fasting literally takes your focus away from physical food and places it on spiritual food. We fast to hear from God and to get closer to Him. How incredible is it that Jesus, who is God, still spent time fasting? When we look at Esther's situation in Esther 4:16, she boldly institutes a fast and then declares that afterward, she will risk her life to go before the king. It was her prayer and fasting that gave her favor before the king. Dear Sister, I truly believe fasting is a powerful spiritual tool that is being underutilized by the body of Christ. Simply put, we do not fast enough, or at all. Fasting is a gift God has given us to bless us with both spiritual and impressive physical benefits.

Recently, several studies have been conducted which show how beneficial fasting is to our physical bodies. Fasting decreases your insulin levels (remember the insulin theory?) which forces your body to burn its own fat to get energy. Yes, you read that correctly, your body will burn its own fat in order to fuel the cells. The lower insulin levels also cause less storage of body fat. These two processes together lead to weight loss! In addition, fasting can lead to amazing mental clarity. When is the last time you felt like taking a test after overindulging in a large meal? Most of the time we want to sleep after eating a large meal because of the large glucose load in our bodies. On the contrary, fasting helps you think more clearly. This is a strategy being used by some of the top Silicon Valley business executives to stay a few steps above the competition. There are also some studies showing that fasting may decrease the risk of certain types of dementia such as Alzheimer's.

You are probably thinking, this all sounds good but won't I starve? That is a good question. And the answer is no. Fasting is different from starving because there is a predetermined endpoint. Your next question may be, won't I feel hungry? The answer to that question is, it depends. The literature on fasting shows that hunger usually comes in waves. Having that knowledge and also knowing the wave will pass can make the fasting time period more tolerable. Most people say they are no longer hungry for the majority of their fasting times once they get used to fasting. Of course, this differs with each person.

Intermittent fasting is different from any diet you could imagine. In fact, it has been said that intermittent fasting is the "undiet." With intermittent fasting, you allow yourself a certain amount of fasting time (drinking only water) each day and a lesser amount of feeding time. A common intermittent fasting method is the 16:8 method, which is fasting for sixteen hours and eating all your calories for the day during an eight hour feeding time. Intermittent fasting fits into your lifestyle and not the other way around. For example, if you have a big dinner party planned, you may choose to fast for breakfast and lunch rather than later in the evening. Or you may not fast at all during that time period and then choose to do a longer fast later on. Fasting gives you freedom. Technically, you can eat whatever you want during your feeding time. Of course, you will see faster results if you adhere to a healthier diet during the feeding time. It also is very important to remember to stay well hydrated when fasting.

I cannot stress enough how powerful fasting can be both as a spiritual and physical tool. For the majority of people, fasting as a lifestyle can produce long-term sustained weight loss and overall improvement in health. Fasting is not advised if you are pregnant or breastfeeding. Also, if you have medical conditions, eating disorders or are taking prescription medications, you should speak with your doctor before beginning a fasting program. There are many people who have been able to be taken off of their medications after starting fasting programs, but you still need to be closely monitored by a physician.

For everyone else, fasting may be the biggest wellness secret of our lifetime. I personally have experienced the benefits of fasting in my life. When I started doing intermittent fasting I had a goal of getting back to my "pre-pregnancy" weight. Not only did I achieve that goal, but I dropped down to my college weight with little effort. I also felt stronger and more focused. I was surprised! I was not counting calories or forcing myself to adhere to a strict diet. All I had to do was avoid eating for certain hours each day. It almost seemed too easy. During my devotion one day, God revealed to me that I was missing out on the spiritual benefits of fasting since my motivation was solely for the health benefits. So now while I'm fasting, I am intentional about feeding my spirit through worship, prayer, and meditating on the Word of God. The change has been remarkable! My vision and purpose have never been clearer and God has been opening doors I could have never imagined. This is why I believe in the power of prayer and fasting. A church that is dedicated to a lifestyle of prayer and fasting will be much healthier than a church that does not focus on this area.

··· Pause & Reflect ···

1. What has been your experience with fasting in the past?

2. How often does your church institute corporate (group) fasts?

3. What issue are you dealing with today that may require fasting in addition to your prayer?

CHAPTER 8

The Discovery

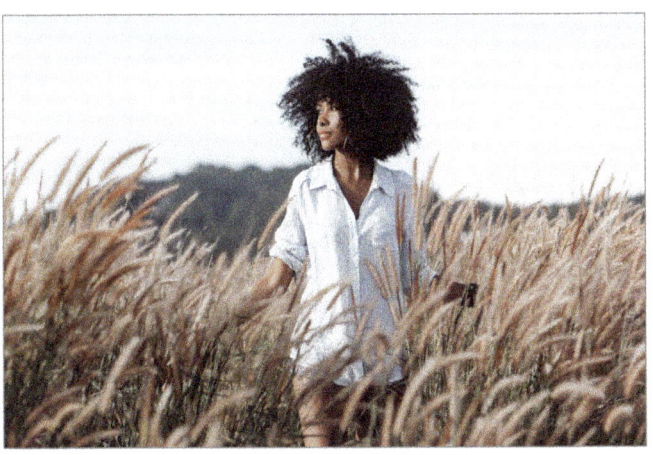

The discovery of worship and wellness begins with understanding who you are in Christ, what God desires for your health and how to use the tools

God has already given you to live your best life. Let us examine each area more closely.

The Call: God chose us long before He formed us within our mother's wombs. Each of us was carefully knit together by God and He recorded each of our days before the first one came to pass. You are not wandering around the world aimlessly. You were placed on this earth for such a time as this. You were also given a mission, one that requires you to place your full trust in God.

Action Steps:

- Make a notecard to place on your bathroom mirror to remind yourself daily that you are handmade by God.

- Spend some time discovering your purpose.

- Take a few moments daily to pray for your "nation."

The Command: God has given each of us a measure of health, for which we will be accountable. Our bodies are not our own and therefore, God commands that we are good stewards of the gift given to us. The truth is, God cares about our health. He cares about our health just as much as He cares about our tithes, our relationships, and our service to others. We must strive for complete wellness—mind, body and soul.

Action Steps:

- ❯ Begin each day with ten minutes of devotion and meditation on the Word of God.
- ❯ Write your daily thoughts in a journal.
- ❯ Make notecards of your affirmations.

The Cause: To live a life that is pleasing to God. God is healing. It was never His desire to see His people suffer from avoidable chronic medical conditions. God's desire is that we live our best health now! Preventing diseases is the way to walk in wellness. We know this has nothing to do with our looks, as we are all made in the image of God. Rather, we keep our bodies healthy as an act of worship to God.

Action Steps:

- Learn your family's health history.

- Visit your primary care physician to be screened for preventable health conditions.

- Improve your diet.

- Consider a lifestyle of fasting, if medically appropriate.

Thank You

Thank you #GEMs (women in this Grace Empowered Movement to reclaim our health) for purchasing and reading this book. I pray it will be the motivation you need to put your health first and to change your mindset in order to achieve any goal you set for yourself. Do not limit yourself. You are stronger than you think. You are smarter than you think. You are more than able to change this world. I am happy to serve as a catalyst. If you found this book to be helpful, please share it with a friend. Do not let what you have read in this book fall to the side. Instead, use these tools to take control of your health and your life. It is time for the church to stand up for our health. Sadly, the majority of the chronic medical conditions that we treat, as physicians, occur due to poor diets and lack of exercise. This has to change! As a Christian and as a physician, it is my mission to share this message with the world. Will you join me? Here's how to connect with me on social media:

FACEBOOK:
www.facebook.com/DrOluchiMD.com

FACEBOOK GROUP:
www.faithandwellnesslifestyle.com

INSTAGRAM:
www.instagram.com/DrOluchiMD/

TWITTER:
www.twitter/DrOluchiMD

LINKEDIN:
www.linkedin.com/in/droluchimd/

Sources

Scriptures marked NASB are taken from the New American Standard Bible®. Copyright © 1960, 1962, 1963, 1968, 1971, 1972, 1973, 1975, 1977, 1995 by The Lockman Foundation. Used by permission.

Scriptures marked NIV are taken from the New International Version®. Copyright © 1973, 1978, 1984, 2011 by Biblica, Inc.™. All rights reserved.

Scriptures marked NKJV are taken from the New King James Version®. Copyright © 1982 by Thomas Nelson. All rights reserved.

Scriptures marked NLT are taken from the New Living Translation®. Copyright © 1996, 2004, 2007, 2013 by Tyndale House Foundation. All rights reserved.

Scriptures marked ISV are taken from *The Holy Bible: International Standard Version*. Release 2.0,

Build 2015.02.09. Copyright © 1995-2014 by ISV Foundation. ALL RIGHTS RESERVED INTERNATIONALLY. Used by permission of Davidson Press, LLC.

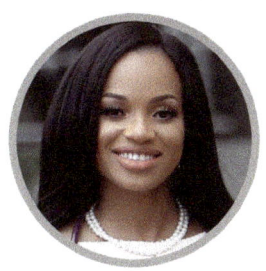

About the Author

Dr. Oluchi Immanuel is a board-certified internal medicine physician, passionate about wellness, disease prevention, faith, and family. Dr. Oluchi was motivated to help women learn about wellness after witnessing her patients deal with the devastating effects of an unhealthy lifestyle. Now, she aims to inspire wellness in every woman at every stage of her life.

Dr. Oluchi attended Iowa State University on a full academic scholarship and graduated with degrees in biology and sociology. She went on to both earn her medical degree and complete her residency at the University of Texas Health Science Center Houston.

Dr. Oluchi is a dynamic speaker, teacher, and social media influencer. Through her videos, webinars, and personalized coaching programs, Dr. Oluchi helps women live their best health now. When she is not working, she enjoys volunteering in her community and spending time with her husband and children.

To learn more, visit her website at www.droluchimd.com

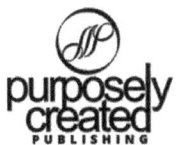

CREATING DISTINCTIVE BOOKS WITH INTENTIONAL RESULTS

We're a collaborative group of creative masterminds with a mission to produce high-quality books to position you for monumental success in the marketplace.

Our professional team of writers, editors, designers, and marketing strategists work closely together to ensure that every detail of your book is a clear representation of the message in your writing.

Want to know more?
Write to us at info@publishyourgift.com
or call (888) 949-6228

Discover great books, exclusive offers, and more at
www.PublishYourGift.com

Connect with us on social media

@publishyourgift

www.ingramcontent.com/pod-product-compliance
Lightning Source LLC
Chambersburg PA
CBHW041958080526
44588CB00021B/2795